CHIROPRACTIC
Pure & Simple

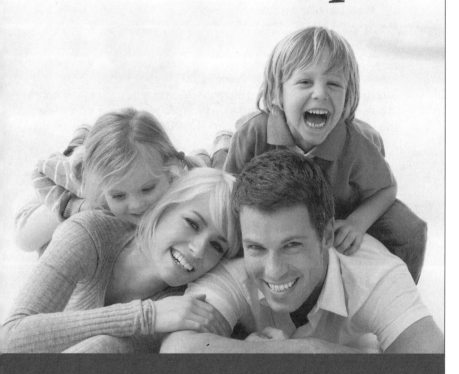

7 WELLNESS SECRETS THAT WILL CHANGE YOUR LIFE

CHIROPRACTIC PURE AND SIMPLE
Seven Wellness Secrets That Will Change Your Life

ISBN: 978-0-615-47994-1

Printed in the United States of America

Cover and Interior Design: Dianna Little
Email: diannalittle@gmail.com

MADDOG PUBLISHING
158 West Caracas Avenue
Hershey, PA 17033
717-533-4840

Disclaimer:
The information contained herein is not intended to be a substitute for medical counseling. It is for informational purposes only and is not intended to diagnose, treat, or cure disease or to take the place of care or treatment by a qualified, licensed health care professional. The opinions expressed are the opinions of the author(s) and most, but not all, are supported by research. Your results will vary. The statements made have not been evaluated by the FDA. Do not alter your medication, start any exercise program, start a diet or in any way alter your health regimen without first consulting your personal physician or other licensed health care professional. Neither the author(s) nor the publisher of this material shall have liability or responsibility to any person or entity with respect to any loss, damage, or injury caused or alleged to be caused directly or indirectly by the advice or information contained in this book.

ACKNOWLEDGEMENTS

I dedicate this book to my best friend, J.C., who has blessed me in more ways than I could have ever thought or imagined.

Secondly, I am forever grateful to my wife, Karen, who is my greatest earthly blessing and the one who deserves most of the credit for my success.

In addition, I want to thank Dr. Tom Horn, Dr. Chris Hood, Dr. Danielle Hood, Dr. James Galgano, Dr. Antonietta Galgano, Dr. Scott Hahn, Dr. Leah Hahn, Dr. Terry Smedstad, Dr. Phil Smith, Dr. Leo McCormick, Dr. Anthony DeMaria, Dr. Bob DeMaria, Dr. Casen DeMaria, Dr. Brian Morris, Dr. Misty Morris, Dr. Jordan Cooper, Dr. Joe Lupo, Dr. Jeff Lupo and Dr. Jessie Lupo for their invaluable contributions.

Dr. John Madeira

TABLE OF

CONTENTS

THE DOCTOR OF THE FUTURE

"The doctor of the future will give no medicine,
but will interest his patients in the care of the human frame,
in diet, and in the cause and prevention of disease."

Attributed to INVENTOR THOMAS A. EDISON

CHIROPRACTIC
PURE & SIMPLE

7 Wellness Secrets That Will Change Your Life

We live at an amazing time in history. Modern medicine and technology continue moving forward by leaps and bounds, unraveling long-held mysteries, and we have made so many amazing forward strides. Improved medicines are being discovered, manufactured and distributed all over the globe each and every day. Cures and treatments for diseases once considered untreatable and deadly are being developed. Less invasive and smarter surgical procedures cut recovery times in half.

Ironically, even with all the advances in modern medicine, we are living in times of unprecedented sickness and poor health. Vast numbers of people suffer from health disorders and disease. According to the U.S. Centers for Disease Control 2010 health statistics report, 48 percent of Americans use at least one prescription drug daily. Thirty-one percent use at least two, and 11 percent take five or more prescriptions daily!

The statistics are staggering. Chronic diseases such as heart disease, cancer and diabetes are responsible for 7 out of 10 deaths among Americans each year and account for 75 percent of all health costs.

Sickness and poor health were never intended to be a part of the American dream, and the cost of treating them threatens to bankrupt us. The U.S. spends well in excess of $1 trillion each year treating sickness and disease with no end in sight. By 2019 that number is expected to grow to $4.48 trillion according to the U.S. Department of Health and Human Services (National Health Expenditures Projections 2009-2019).

Most of our medical advancements, as wonderful as they are, have been directed at treating illness, not preventing it. What we really need is more emphasis on improving and maintaining our health, not just new and more expensive ways to treat it. This is even more compelling when you consider that nearly 80 percent of the top ten causes of death are entirely preventable.

We live with very high levels of stress. The food we eat is too often highly processed and void of healthy nutrients. We do not exercise often enough nor get adequate rest compared to previous generations. The human costs of pain and suffering and the toll on our quality of life is astonishing. People with vibrant health and a high quality of life are the exception to the rule.

The good news is that understanding seven simple but profound health secrets can prevent most of the sickness and deaths that occur every day. Teaching those secrets and arming you with that knowledge is what this book is all about.

1

"A Healthy Spine Equals a Healthier You"

Your spine is directly connected to the function of every part of your body. When your spine is healthy, your body simply functions better. When properly aligned, fed, rested, exercised and maintained, the human body has an amazing ability to heal and repair itself without any conscious or outside help. Your spine is the key player in your body's natural ability to heal and to maintain itself.

As a natural health care provider who specializes in wellness, I believe that the medical community needs to focus more on health enhancement and sickness prevention rather than on treating illness. It is so much easier to stay healthy than it is to get healthy once you are sick, especially after you have been diagnosed with a serious disease. If we were to encourage people to do more to stay healthy and enhance their body's own natural ability to heal, there would be much less sickness in the world. It makes sense from an economic standpoint, too. Our grandmothers understood this concept years ago when they said, "An ounce of prevention is worth a pound of cure."

The body's incredible ability to heal is controlled by your nervous system, a system so powerful that it controls every function in your body from breathing to blinking to thinking, moving and the beating of your heart. Every function of your body obeys the nervous system, which consists of three parts:

1. The brain, the supercomputer of the body,
2. The spinal cord, which runs inside your spine and is connected to the brain. This "super-highway" carries nerve impulses from the brain to the rest of the body via....
3. The nerve network, which carries nerve impulses (messages) from the spinal cord out to every cell, tissue and organ in the body.

The brain controls your body much like a conductor directs an orchestra, instructing each "instrument" when and how to perform. It is the brain's job to keep the body healthy and all its parts functioning in perfect harmony. When the body gets sick, the brain initiates self-repair by sending messages down the spinal cord and out over the nerve network. The messages are actually minute electrical nerve impulses that instruct the body where to send fresh, oxygenated blood, extra nutrients, white blood cells, and new building materials to repair any sickness or injury quickly and completely. These repairs begin to occur without our conscious knowledge often long before any symptoms ever surface.

Your spine is composed of 24 individual spinal bones called vertebrae and is a magnificent feat of engineering. The spinal bones are able to move and bend, allowing you to twist and turn your body freely. Unfortunately, the spinal bones can become misaligned quite easily. This happens to most everyone at one time or another from such varied causes as sports injuries, car accidents, and slips and falls.

When a spinal bone shifts out of its normal position, chiropractors call it a "subluxation," which literally means "a minor dislocation." When a spinal bone becomes misaligned, the opening where the nerve exits the spine becomes smaller. This crowds and squeezes the nerve as it passes through the opening. Over time the nerve becomes irritated and the proper flow of electrical nerve impulses becomes blocked. Instead of 100 percent nerve flow traveling from the brain over the nerve to the body, the electrical nerve signals become weakened. The result is much like a dimmer switch dims a light fixture in your home. This interruption in nerve flow is called "nerve interference" and is one of the key reasons many healthy people can become sick. Nerve interference blocks the nerve messages going to and from the affected body part which opens the door for sickness, pain or poor function to develop there. Once

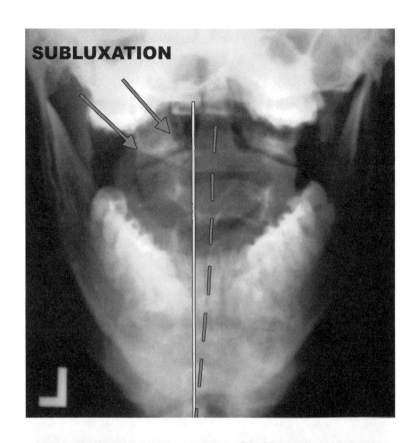

SUBLUXATION

CAUSES OF SUBLUXATIONS	
(spinal misalignments)	

- Improper lifting
- Trauma to a baby's upper neck during the birth process
- Sports impacts and injuries
- Unhealthy sleeping positions
- Poor posture

- Car accidents
- Falls while learning to walk
- Falls on slippery surfaces
- Repetitive activities such as assembly line work, sitting at computers
- Prolonged stress

sickness or disease sets in, nerve interference also makes it much more difficult for the body to heal itself.

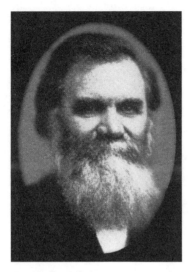

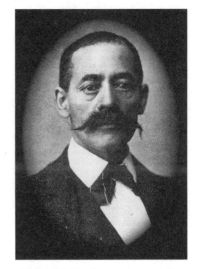

Dr. D. D. Palmer   *Harvey Lillard*

Nearly everyone has experienced tens if not hundreds of impacts to their body in their lifetime, which explains why subluxations are very widespread. Ninety percent of the population walks around with one or more misalignments in their spine without their knowledge. Most subluxations go unnoticed because they most often do not cause any symptoms directly at the spine. Because subluxations are so prevalent and occur early in life from birth trauma and from nearly 1500 falls while learning to walk, every person's spine should be checked for subluxations.

Dr. Daniel David Palmer, the world's first chiropractor, coined the term "subluxation". Chiropractic was discovered in 1895 when patient Harvey Lillard's hearing was completely restored after receiving the world's first chiropractic adjustment from Dr. Palmer in Davenport, Iowa. Since that time chiropractic has become the largest natural healing profession in the world and is one of the fastest growing health care professions. There are an estimated 70,000 practicing chiropractors throughout the world today.

It is the role of the chiropractor to check the spine for subluxations and to correct them. A friend of Dr. Palmer, Reverend Samuel Weed, named chiropractic. It means health care "done by hand." Chiropractic treatments are called "spinal adjustments." Spinal adjustment is a term used to describe a chiropractic manipulation designed to gently push a misaligned spinal bone back toward its proper position. Spinal adjustments are normally painless and are usually done by hand or with the assistance of an adjusting instrument.

Chiropractic care is very safe, comfortable and effective. It has been estimated that 1,000,000 spinal adjustments are given worldwide every single day. The safety of chiropractic care is confirmed by the low malpractice insurance premiums that chiropractors pay compared to the often enormous fees paid by medical physicians and surgeons. This high degree of safety is due in part to a thorough examination process that normally includes a detailed consultation, examination and most often includes taking x-rays of the spine. The x-ray pictures help the doctor to determine the degree and severity of misalignments in the spine and to see if there are any complicating factors such as arthritis or spinal curvatures contributing to the problem.

Chiropractors today are very well educated and receive eight years of combined undergraduate and graduate education at

18 chiropractic institutions around the world. Upon graduation they are awarded a Doctor of Chiropractic degree (abbreviated "D.C."). Chiropractors must pass rigorous national board examinations and licensure requirements. They are licensed in all 50 U.S. states and nearly every developed country worldwide.

Correcting a spine takes time. Think orthodontics for the spine. Normal timeframes to return a spine back to its optimum position can take anywhere from 6-18 months for the average adult, less for infants and children. If that seems like a long time, it's not. Just a few short years ago, before current advances in research and technology, it took twice as long with less correction possible. Today's chiropractic patients are the grateful recipients of years of chiropractic research, discovery and steady improvement in chiropractic care.

Having subluxations in your spine can be very serious. Subluxations are the doorways to many kinds of health disorders because they hinder the brain's ability to direct function, healing and repair.

This is a brief list of common health problems that can be directly or indirectly caused by spinal misalignments:

- Back pain
- Headaches
- Migraines
- Neck pain

- Spinal curvature
- Asthma
- Allergies
- Sinus problems
- Chronic colds
- Lowered immune resistance
- Arthritis
- Fibromyalgia
- Joint pain
- Poor posture
- Difficulty sleeping
- Lack of energy
- Digestive difficulty
- Hip and leg pain
- Carpal tunnel syndrome
- Sleepy arms and hands
- Plus many more!

Many people suffering from countless health disorders could be helped if their spines were checked and corrected. People often struggle with all types of sickness and maladies without ever considering that the root of their health problem(s) may be the result of a misalignment affecting the normal and proper function of the nerves exiting their spine.

A well-aligned spine is vital to your good health. Every member of the family needs to have their spine checked. No other health care provider is trained or qualified to check for subluxations. If you are not currently seeing a chiropractor or have never had your spine checked, I urge you to do so as soon as possible.

New research continually confirms the benefits of spinal care. You will never experience complete health and healing in your body apart from a fully functioning spine and nervous system. Your body will thank you with more vibrant health, renewed healing ability and a higher quality of life.

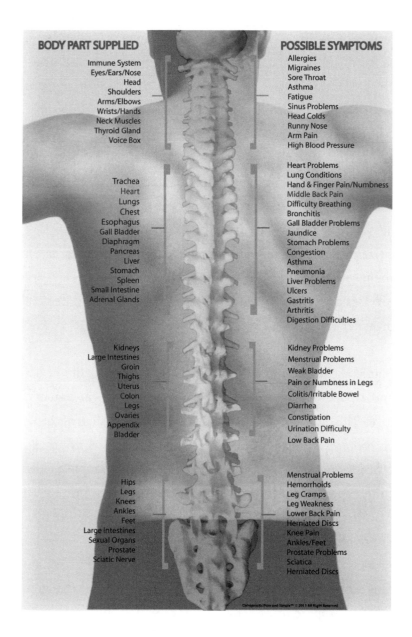

BODY PART SUPPLIED	POSSIBLE SYMPTOMS
Immune System	Allergies
Eyes/Ears/Nose	Migraines
Head	Sore Throat
Shoulders	Asthma
Arms/Elbows	Fatigue
Wrists/Hands	Sinus Problems
Neck Muscles	Head Colds
Thyroid Gland	Runny Nose
Voice Box	Arm Pain
	High Blood Pressure
	Heart Problems
	Lung Conditions
Trachea	Hand & Finger Pain/Numbness
Heart	Middle Back Pain
Lungs	Difficulty Breathing
Chest	Bronchitis
Esophagus	Gall Bladder Problems
Gall Bladder	Jaundice
Diaphragm	Stomach Problems
Pancreas	Congestion
Liver	Asthma
Stomach	Pneumonia
Spleen	Liver Problems
Small Intestine	Ulcers
Adrenal Glands	Gastritis
	Arthritis
	Digestion Difficulties
Kidneys	Kidney Problems
Large Intestines	Menstrual Problems
Groin	Weak Bladder
Thighs	Pain or Numbness in Legs
Uterus	Colitis/Irritable Bowel
Colon	Diarrhea
Legs	Constipation
Ovaries	Urination Difficulty
Appendix	Low Back Pain
Bladder	
	Menstrual Problems
Hips	Hemorrhoids
Legs	Leg Cramps
Knees	Leg Weakness
Ankles	Lower Back Pain
Feet	Herniated Discs
Large Intestines	Knee Pain
Sexual Organs	Ankles/Feet
Prostate	Prostate Problems
Sciatic Nerve	Sciatica
	Herniated Discs

So what does current research say about chiropractic care? According to the Journal of Vertebral Subluxation Research, more than 40 studies have shown that chiropractic care results in statistically significant improvements in breathing, range of motion, heart rate, glandular function, cardiovascular function, immune function, muscle strength, athletic ability, reaction times, brain function, information processing, and healing and recovery times.

Rupert, Manello and Sandefur stated that chiropractic patients over 65 years of age who received chiropractic wellness care for five years or longer (when compared to U.S. citizens of the same age not receiving chiropractic care), spent only 31 percent of the national average for health care services and experienced a 50 percent reduction in medical provider visits.

Blanks, Schuster and Dobson investigated the quality of life and wellness of people who regularly receive chiropractic care. This study, the largest of its kind, consisted of 2,818 chiropractic patients attending 156 different chiropractic offices. An overwhelming 95 percent of the people in the study reported a strong, direct connection between receiving chiropractic care and experiencing a healthy, more active, improved quality of life.

The Chiropractic Research Journal reported on a review of 45 chiropractic research studies, 5 case studies and 23 scientific review articles and concluded that chiropractic adjustments are proven to enhance the health of the body, which included: decreasing blood pressure, reducing the ill effects of asthma, increasing the numbers of T cells (immune cells) in the body, relieving the symptoms of osteoarthritis, enhancing immune function in certain white blood cells and even urinary function.

The American Medical Association and WebMD reported recently on a study comparing four years of consecutive health care coverage for more than 700,000 health plan members. The study concluded that when a health insurance plan includes coverage for chiropractic services, there is a significantly lower need for medical surgeries, hospitalizations and other medical treatments. In addition, when a health insurance plan includes chiropractic care as a covered service, it cut the cost of treating back pain by 28 percent, reduced hospitalization among back pain patients by 41 percent, decreased back surgeries by 32 percent and reduced the cost of medical imaging (such as MRI and x-rays) by 37 percent.

Lastly, the Journal of Manipulative and Physiological Therapeutics reported that chiropractic adjustments do more than just provide relief for neck and back pain and increase range of motion. To find out exactly what other non-pain related wellness benefits people receive from chiropractic care, they distributed 1504 questionnaires to people who had just received a chiropractic adjustment. The patients reported experiencing easier breathing, improved digestion, clearer/sharper vision, improved circulation, less ringing in their ears, reduced acne/eczema and fewer symptoms of asthma and allergies.

Current research and scientific study will continue to discover both how and why chiropractic and other types of natural care are so effective in enhancing our health and well being. Each of the remaining chapters will explore the six other wellness secrets that play a huge role in improving the quality of your life by enhancing your body's own inherent, natural healing ability.

"Real Food Really Matters"

Y ou have heard people say, "You are what you eat." A more truthful statement, however, is "You *become* what you eat." Let me explain. Your body is made up of trillions of individual cells, each of which needs to be fed. The food you put in your mouth today becomes the building material your body uses tomorrow to replace, repair and regenerate every single cell in your body. So what you eat each day has a huge impact on your future health.

Because most of your cells only last three to six months before dying and being replaced, you have an entirely new body once or twice a year! That's encouraging news, because just a few months of making wise food choices can make a marked difference in your level of health.

Think of it this way: If you were going to build a house in a tornado or hurricane zone, would you want to build it out of wooden two by fours or would you rather it be made out of cinder blocks and cement? Do you remember the story of the three little pigs and the big bad wolf? "I'll huff and I'll puff and I'll blow your house down!" Of course you would build a brick house not one made out of hay and stubble. In much the same way, what you eat each day is the building material that will be used to construct either strong cells inside in your body or weak, sickly ones. When a tornado or hurricane (sickness or disease) comes knocking at your door, you can be at peace knowing your house (your health) has been built to withstand it.

Foods either build your body up or tear it down; they are either constructive or destructive. If you consistently eat constructive foods that provide what your body needs to build strong, vibrant cells, you will experience improved health and all its benefits. Conversely, if you feed your body soda, candy bars, potato chips and donuts on a regular basis, your cells are being built with second- or third-rate building materials, and you are setting yourself up for disease and poor health over time.

Eating more fruits and vegetables has been strongly linked to better health. The results of a recent University of Oxford study showed that increasing fruit and vegetable intake can reduce your risk of dying from heart disease. The findings, which were published in the *European Heart Journal* (reported January 19, 2011), revealed that those who ate eight servings of fruits and vegetables a day had a 22 percent lower risk of fatal heart disease compared with those consuming less than three portions a day.

Researchers at the Harvard School of Public Health are studying the diets of more than 83,000 women who entered the Nurses' Health Study in 1980. One of the key findings so far is that pre-menopausal women who consumed at least five servings of fruits and vegetables per day had a 70 percent lower risk of developing breast cancer compared with those that consumed less than two servings per day. Even more surprising is that the women involved in this study had an immediate family member with breast cancer, which would increase their genetic risk of developing cancer themselves. The consumption of fruits and vegetables has the power to overrule the genetic component of cancer development.

The problem in our fast food world is that the average person gets only three or fewer servings of fruits or vegetables in their daily diet. Ironically, it is not that hard to increase to five to eight servings or more per day. Simply topping your morning cereal with a cup of blueberries, enjoying an apple, orange or banana for a mid-morning snack and eating a field greens salad for lunch topped with carrots, tomatoes or radishes quickly increases your servings — and by just noon! Have some green beans, carrots, broccoli, cauliflower, peas or lima beans at dinner and you have reached six servings. For dessert enjoy a large bowl of strawberries or raspberries with whipped cream and you have reached eight. It is really that easy!

With so many restaurants (who are more than willing to super-size your order for an extra twenty-five cents), eating an unhealthy diet has never been so easy...or so dangerous. Fortunately, public demand is beginning to change the menus at some of the most popular fast food restaurants to include salads and fruit. Even so, their menus are dominated by dead foods that are high in calories, saturated fat, chemical additives and low in nutritional value.

Our first rule for healthy eating is to eat "live foods" instead of "dead foods."

Examples of live foods include eggs, fresh lean cuts of meat, and fruits and vegetables. Vegetables are especially important because they contain a rich mix of vitamins, minerals, enzymes and naturally occurring cancer fighting compounds. They also contain minimal calories so you can eat them in abundance without worrying about your waistline!

Dead foods are processed foods, typically made in a manufacturing plant and most often packaged in a box, can or mechanically sealed wrapper. Examples include most breakfast cereals, candy, cakes and pies, trans fat oils (which are known to be cancer causing and normally labeled as "partially hydrogenated oils"), most frozen prepared meals, and canned fruits and vegetables. The ingredient lists of these dead foods usually include a long list of chemical preservatives, food additives, artificial flavors, food colorings and words that most of us cannot even pronounce. This leads us to a good second rule to follow when making healthier food choices.

Our second rule: If you can't pronounce it, you probably shouldn't eat it!

A third guideline to follow when choosing to eat a healthier diet is that the shorter the ingredients list, the healthier a food is for you. Becoming a label reader will help you to make healthier food choices. Today's food labels provide great information about ingredients and nutritional content. Imagine you are buying a loaf of bread at the grocery store. You avoid the white bread because you know that white bread is not as good for you as wheat bread because it is more heavily processed. Good first step!

But which wheat bread should you buy? You pick up two loaves of wheat bread and scan the ingredients lists. One says "whole wheat flour" as the first ingredient and the other says, "enriched wheat." What's the difference? "Whole wheat flour" includes the entire wheat kernel and all the nutrients that naturally occur in wheat, including the fiber and micronutrients. The natural color of the wheat kernel contributes to the brown coloring of the bread.

"Enriched wheat flour," on the other hand, contains mainly "enriched" white flour. Only part of the wheat kernel is used. This flour has to be enriched to replace the major nutrients lost during the flour milling process. The vitamins put back into it are often synthetic vitamins because they are less expensive than their healthier, naturally occurring cousins.

The brown color of the bread is a result of added food colorings or molasses to make it appear healthier.

Continuing your examination of the ingredients lists, you notice that one list is much longer than the other. It contains words like "glucose" and "dextrose" — both of which are forms of refined sugar. Also included on the list is water, high fructose corn syrup (a controversial form of liquid sugar), cultured wheat starch, wheat bran (added fiber), partially hydrogenated soybean oil (the name for trans fat) and dough conditioners.

The shorter list looks like this: whole-wheat flour, water, wheat gluten, honey, oats, yeast, salt. This loaf is the winner by a long shot because generally speaking the shorter the ingredients list, the less additives are in the food product, and the less processed and the healthier it is for you.

Therefore, our third rule for healthier eating is: Foods with shorter ingredients lists are healthier for you.

Simply stated, excellent health comes from the choices we routinely make every day. This includes a steady, conscious decision to eat foods that will build you up on the inside (constructive foods), not tear you down (destructive foods). Most foods, beverages and snacks fall into one of these two categories, so it is a good idea to always consider, "Is this food going to build me up on the inside or will it tear me down?" You simply cannot feed your body a steady diet of destructive foods and beverages and expect it to be able to fend off illness and battle disease when they come knocking at your door.

Our discussion of a healthier diet would not be complete without addressing the beverages we consume. Good old fashioned water is still the best beverage to drink. Compare that with soda, which routinely contains the equivalent of 17 packets of white sugar per 20 ounce bottle. "So what's the big deal?" you ask. Many experts believe that sugary sodas and beverages are the number one cause of diabetes, the fastest growing disease in developed countries. I agree.

Sugar also makes you fat, steals your energy and causes inflammation in your joints. Stop drinking sugar-based beverages, replace them with water for 90 days and see what happens. Many of my patients who accept this challenge lose ten to fifteen pounds in 90 days. Many report their energy levels improve significantly, their joint pain gets better, and the frequency and intensity of their chronic headaches decrease or they disappear completely!

It should be noted that diet soda and diet drinks have an entirely different set of problems due to their chemical sweeteners. Artificial sweeteners are suspected of being a potential cause of Alzheimer's disease and dementia. There is also research that suggests that changing from regular soda to diet soda does not cause you to lose weight; in fact, some evidence suggests that they lead to greater weight gain.

Many foods have healthy sounding names like "fruit bits," "fruit rolls" or "fruit snacks," but they are really candy made mainly of sugar with small amounts of added fruit juice. For example, this is the ingredients list for a popular strawberry flavored fruit rolled candy. Based on what we have learned so far, you decide if this is a healthy food or not, and whether it is something that you really want your kids or grandkids to be eating:

Strawberry Ingredients: Pears From Concentrate, Corn Syrup, Dried Corn Syrup, Sugar, Partially Hydrogenated Cottonseed Oil, Citric Acid, Sodium Citrate, Acetylated Mono And Diglycerides, Pectin, Malic Acid, Natural Flavor, Vitamin C (Ascorbic Acid), Color (Red 40, Yellows 5, 6, Blue 1).

While we are on the subject of feeding our children and we are taking tests, see what you think about this. Here is the ingredients list for a very popular fast food chain's chicken nuggets for children:

White boneless chicken, water, food starch-modified, salt, seasoning [yeast extract, salt, wheat starch, natural flavoring (botanical source), safflower oil, dextrose, citric acid], sodium phosphate, natural flavor (botanical source). Battered and breaded with: water, enriched flour (bleached wheat flour, niacin, reduced iron, thiamin mononitrate,

continued

riboflavin, folic acid), yellow corn flour, bleached wheat flour, food starch-modified, salt, leavening (baking soda, sodium acid pyrophosphate, sodium aluminum phosphate, mono-calcium phosphate, calcium lactate), spices, wheat starch, dextrose, corn starch. Prepared in vegetable oil (Canola oil, corn oil, soybean oil, hydrogenated soybean oil with TBHQ and citric acid added to preserve freshness). Dimethylpolysiloxane added as an antifoaming agent.

Does that sound like chicken to you? If this fast food company would make these chicken nuggets from real food ingredients, the list would look more like this:

Organic chicken, organic bread crumbs (organic wheat, flour, yeast, organic expeller pressed palm oil, salt), cooking oil.

Finally, we need more fiber in our diets. Today's nutrition experts recommend eating more whole grains, fruits and vegetables to increase dietary fiber. Only 25 percent of Americans get the necessary daily amount of fiber in their diets. Not getting enough fiber is one of the main reasons why so many people suffer from constipation, lack of energy and high cholesterol. Much of the colon cancer in this country is an indirect result of insufficient fiber intake. Diets that include high fiber foods (fruits, vegetables, nuts, whole grains) help reduce the risk of some types of cancers and help lower bad cholesterol levels, too.

So you can now see that Wellness Secret 2 "Real Food Really Matters" is a major piece of the wellness formula. Getting your spine in the healthiest shape possible and eating healthy, constructive foods will help you enjoy a longer, more vibrant life. Let's take a look at Wellness Secret 3!

Wellness Action Steps

1. You become what you eat, so choose to eat healthier food and beverages.
2. Eat more "live" foods and eat less "dead" foods.
3. If you can't pronounce it, don't eat it!
4. Foods with shorter ingredients lists are healthier for you.
5. Eat 5-8 servings of fresh fruits or vegetables per day.
6. Eliminate sugar (especially white sugar) and artificial sweeteners from your diet.
7. Drink more water and fewer sugary beverages.
8. Start reading food labels so you know what you are eating.
9. Get more fiber in your diet.
10. Do not eat food that contains trans fat oils (partially hydrogenated oils).

"Just Say 'No' to Sweets"

Most people have been taught that sugar is bad for their teeth, but the negative effects of sweets on your overall health go far beyond that beautiful smile of yours. Plainly stated, the sugar in sweets is the precursor to many health problems, which gradually accumulate over time.

When I speak of sugar, I am not talking about naturally occurring sweeteners such as honey, real maple syrup, stevia or agave nectar. I am talking about the white refined sugar commonly sold in 5-pound bags that comes from sugar cane and sugar beets. Refined white sugar is the result of a complex refining process that includes bleaching. This type of sugar is added to almost all processed foods.

Most people think they do not eat much sugar but we get more sugar in our diets than we realize. The average American in the 1700s ate the equivalent of one 5-pound bag of white sugar per year. Today that number has skyrocketed to thirty 5-pound bags (150 pounds) — plus an additional 20 pounds of controversial liquid corn sweeteners annually. That is a whole bunch of sugar, and it's no wonder America is getting fat! White sugar is added to all kinds of foods and beverages, and if you were not checking the labels you would never realize it.

White refined sugar is a leading contributor to almost all major diseases, especially diabetes, arthritis, heart disease and obesity. Food manufacturers sneak it into foods all the time without our knowledge.

I am not suggesting that an occasional piece of cake or a candy bar will have a huge and immediate negative impact on your health. But regular daily consumption of sugar will compromise your health, because your body does not recognize white sugar as a real food. Become a label reader and begin avoiding foods that contain added sugars. Some of the more common names for hidden sugars seen on food labels include: dextrose, high fructose corn syrup, lactose, maltose, maltodextrin, sucrose, galactose, fructose, barley malt, evaporated cane juice, corn syrup, corn sweetener and rice syrup.

Sugar is in nearly everything that we eat. It is in alcohol, ketchup, candy, soda, desserts, fruit juices, wine, beer, bread, most processed foods, and the list could continue on and on. Even if you throw away all the white sugar in your house (and I suggest that you do) and never buy it again, chances are highly probable that you will still consume sugar, especially if you eat processed foods or regularly eat at restaurants.

What does sugar actually do to the body? The main problem is that sugar puts a strain on the immune system, the system that protects the body from sickness and disease. Sugar intake causes the pancreas to secrete abnormal amounts of insulin, which is required to break the sugar down. Insulin causes the cells in the body to store the sugar in the form of fat. This simple process explains why America has such an obesity epidemic. High sugar consumption is making Americans the fattest people on earth while raising the rate of diabetes to epidemic proportions.

In addition, after the cells in the body have metabolized the sugar, the insulin still remains in the blood. And when insulin stays in the blood past its expiration time, it hinders the release of growth hormones. As a result, children who consume large amounts of sugar are at risk of growth hormone deficiency that can have a negative impact on their body's overall growth. This is not to mention the all too obvious behavioral problems commonly seen in children whose diets are high in sugary, processed foods.

Nancy Appleton, author of *Lick the Sugar Habit*, lists 76 ways that sugar can ruin your health. Here are just a few:

1. Sweets can suppress your immune system and impair your defenses against infectious disease.
2. Sweets can produce a significant increase in your overall cholesterol, raise triglycerides (blood fats), escalate bad cholesterol and decrease good cholesterol.

3. Sweets feed cancer cells and have been connected with the development of cancer of the breast, ovaries, prostate, rectum, pancreas, biliary tract, lung, gallbladder and stomach.
4. Sweets can increase fasting levels of glucose and can cause hypoglycemia.
5. Sweets can weaken eyesight.
6. Sweets can cause premature aging and wrinkling of the skin.
7. Daily consumption of sweets causes weight gain, which often leads to obesity.
8. Sweets can cause or aggravate autoimmune diseases such as arthritis, asthma and multiple sclerosis.
9. Sweets can cause headaches, including migraines.
10. Sweets are addictive because sugar is addictive.

As bad as sugary, sweet foods are for you, many wellness experts believe that artificial sweeteners are even worse. It has been suggested that artificial chemical sweeteners may cause Alzheimer's and dementia if consumed in large quantities.

Sugar is not food; it acts more like a chemical or a drug in your body. That should be reason enough to eliminate or greatly reduce sugar from your diet. When you do, you will enjoy increased energy, more normal cholesterol levels, diminished aches and pains and weight loss — among many other health benefits.

"Get Your Daily ZZZs"

While much attention is given to the healthful benefits of a good diet and correct nutrition, proper rest is an equally important part of good health. Some people consider sleep "optional," but that could not be further from the truth. If you want to have extraordinary health, superior mental performance and to feel your best each day, sleep is an absolute necessity, not a luxury. Every night you plug your cell phone into its "recharger" so it is ready to function correctly the next day. In the same way, consider the proper amount of quality sleep the "recharger" for your body.

Sleep needs vary from person to person, but most experts agree that adults need between seven to eight hours of sleep each night. School-age children and teens need nine hours of sleep each night. Pre-school age children typically sleep between ten to twelve hours per day, and newborns sleep between sixteen and eighteen hours per day.

Adults sleep in cycles of approximately 90 minutes. Each cycle includes a period of light sleep that gradually leads to very deep sleep and then back again. We have all experienced the "punch-drunk" disoriented feeling that results from being awakened during the deepest part of our sleep. If circumstances regularly prevent us from entering the deepest part of our sleep cycles, we are unable to get the deep sleep required to feel fully rested.

During periods of sleep, your body repairs itself, reversing the effects of aging and the stresses and strains of your busy life. Studies show that most people do not get adequate sleep. It is not just the amount that matters, but also the quality of sleep that most profoundly affects its healthful benefits.

Skimping on sleep has a price. Lack of sleep affects mood, personal performance, can make you feel irritable, is linked to poor behavior in children and increases the likelihood of depression in adults. It also impacts your ability to make good decisions and drastically increases the likelihood of car accidents and industrial injuries. Those who are regularly deprived of restful sleep are also at increased risk for high blood pressure and heart disease, as well as other medical conditions.

Deep sleep is important to healing. The deeper sleep cycles trigger the release of growth hormone, which fuels growth in children, builds muscle, slows the aging process and enhances healing and repair on a cellular level in all age groups. Inadequate levels of growth hormone are linked to obesity, diabetes and sugar and carbohydrate cravings.

Dreaming is also an important part of restful sleep. Even if you are unable to remember your dreams, sleep scientists confirm that we all dream. Dreams are accompanied by rapid eye movements known as REM sleep, and dreaming seems to be important to our health. Experiments in which subjects are deprived of the dreaming cycle of sleep suffer from irritability and poor judgment.

We need sleep to think clearly and to be able to react quickly. The pathways that help us to learn and remember are very active while we are sleeping, too. Research strongly suggests that people who are taught mentally challenging tasks do much better after a good night's rest. One of the best ways to prepare for a big presentation at work or an important test at school is to get a full night of sleep the night before.

If you don't sleep well, try the following suggestions:

- Go to bed at a consistent bedtime each evening.
- Cut caffeine and nicotine out of your life.
- Avoid alcohol before bedtime.
- Avoid eating late at night.
- Abstain from drinking liquids after 7pm.
- Avoid taking medications that may disrupt your sleep.
- Take a hot bath before bedtime to help you to relax.

- Read a book or magazine at or before bedtime to help you unwind.

The environment can impact the quality of your sleep as well. One of the most important and overlooked ways to improve your sleep is to buy a new, comfortable mattress. Make sure you have a pillow that properly supports your head and upper spine, especially your neck. Reduce the temperature of your bedroom and remove anything that distracts or disrupts your sleep. Intense outdoor lights, bright alarm clocks, flashing light and noise from televisions and computers can affect your ability to get a full night's rest.

Some people find it helpful to sleep while listening to noise machines that drown out other background sounds. These devices generally offer a multitude of options, such as waves crashing on the beach, birds chirping, rainfall or white noise (soft static).

Do your best to shut off your mind at bedtime by reading an enjoyable book or a magazine for a few minutes after you get into bed. This can help keep you from focusing on the worry, fear and concerns that so often come to the forefront of our minds once our day comes to a close and we climb into bed.

Finally, forgiving those who have hurt you, mending bad relationships, and reducing your personal stress levels can help you tremendously to get more peaceful, undisturbed sleep.

"Stress Less"

Stress is defined as a force that strains or deforms. It can also be defined as a force that puts unnecessary and unhealthy strain on our minds and our bodies that ultimately affects our health in a negative way. Your body's reaction to stress is meant to protect you, but when your body is constantly fighting the effects of stress, your health can pay a high price.

Our bodies are wired to react to stress in ways meant to protect us from threats from predators and other dangerous circumstances. But when we are constantly feeling stressed and on edge, that fight-or-flight reaction stays turned on. The resulting overexposure to adrenaline, cortisol and other stress hormones affects nearly every physical process in your body. This puts you at increased risk for numerous health problems.

No one is exempt from stress. Of the three main kinds of stress, physical stress is the most obvious. You can get physically stressed from straining to lift something that is too heavy.

You can get physical stress from an impact to your body due to a sports injury or car accident, from repetitive work on an assembly line, slumping over a computer all day or continually working grueling hours. These stresses are physical because they are most easily detected in our physical bodies.

Chemical stress is another form of stress that occurs when chemicals in the form of prescription drugs, cigarette smoke, alcohol, and other airborne or food-based pollutants or toxins get into our systems and alter their ability to perform optimally. This kind of stress is the most subtle kind of all because it often accumulates slowly over time and is not always easy to detect.

The third type of stress is emotional or mental stress, which can be equally deadly because it typically builds slowly over time without our awareness. You have probably heard the story of the frog in the pot that did not realize he was being boiled to death because he didn't notice the temperature of his environment gradually rising. Don't become that frog! Emotional/mental stress may not always be easily seen or felt in its early stages. Financial difficulties, the responsibilities of being a single parent or caring for a parent with dementia are all examples of emotional and mental stress that can build gradually over time and become very intense.

Regardless of the type, all stress will have negative long-term effects on our health if not recognized and dealt with. Stress can conceal itself for years and then all of a sudden have drastic consequences in your seemingly healthy life when it manifests as an unexpected heart attack, stroke, high blood pressure or cancer diagnosis.

Many experts believe that the majority of our health problems are either directly or indirectly linked to stress. The American Institute of Stress of the American Psychological Association states that stress is directly or indirectly linked to the six leading causes of death. They also state that more than 50 percent of adults suffer from its adverse effects and that $300 billion is spent annually on medical costs related to stress.

What are the effects of stress on your health? Stress impacts not only your physical health but also your moods and behavior. The following chart lists some of the more common effects of long-term stress in these three areas:

COMMON EFFECTS OF STRESS		
On your body	**On your mood**	**On your behavior**
• Headaches • Muscle Tension • Joint Pain • Chest Pain • Fatigue • Loss of Sex Drive • Sexual/Erectile Dysfunction • Digestive Upset • Difficulty Sleeping	• Anxiety • Restlessness • Lack of Motivation or Focus • Irritability or Anger • Sadness or Depression	• Over Eating or Under Eating • Anger Outbursts • Drug and/or Alcohol Abuse • Tobacco Use • Social Withdrawal • Depression • Anxiety

SOURCE: American Psychological Association's "Stress in America" 2010

Our bodies are actually designed to tolerate quite a bit of stress, and that is good news. Though we may never be able to totally eliminate stress and its negative effects completely, we can definitely limit its grip on us. The answer to stress is not trying to rid our lives of it but recognizing and keeping a handle on it.

Here are a dozen tips to help you minimize stress and be more content with your life:

1. Make time for more fun because laughter is really good medicine.
2. Stop worrying, because 95 percent of the things we worry about never happen.
3. Stop comparing yourself or your life with others. Doing so is always a "no win" proposition.
4. Remain grateful for everything that is good about your life so you can feel better about the things that are not.
5. Stop worrying about what other people think. How you feel is the only thing that really matters.
6. Get to bed early each night and exercise regularly because it is known to reduce the effects of stress on our bodies.
7. Go on more vacations. We all need regular breaks from our daily routine.
8. Get regular massages to reduce the muscular tension that accumulates in your body from stress.

9. Purge negative people and their negative attitudes from your life and replace them with the happy, smiling kind.
10. Allow more margin in your daily schedule so you don't feel so rushed.
11. De-clutter your environment.
12. See your chiropractor regularly to help your body function at its best and lessen the effects of stress.

Though we can never get rid of all our stress, practicing the **Seven Wellness Secrets** will greatly reduce the negative effects of stress on your health. Always remember that your health is your single greatest asset and that without it nothing else matters very much. Do not let stress destroy your plans to live a long and wonderful life.

WELLNESS SECRET

6

"Keep Moving"

One of the common denominators among the healthiest people is consistent exercise. Exercise and wellness go hand in hand and have so many obvious benefits. Vigorous physical activity improves your sleep, decreases the effects of stress, burns unwanted calories, raises metabolism, improves digestion, and increases the speed of food traveling through the digestive system. It helps flush your lymphatic system, eliminating wastes and toxins from the body more quickly and efficiently.

Inactivity poses as great a health risk as smoking, contributing to heart disease, diabetes, weight gain, high blood pressure, cancer, depression, arthritis and osteoporosis. The statistics are astounding as to how many Americans get little to no exercise at all. The Centers for Disease Control and Prevention reported that 36 percent of U.S. adults did not engage in any leisure-time physical activity in 2008.

So start where you are and get moving! Any amount of exercise is good for you! Start stretching on the side of your bed each morning or do a calisthenics routine that includes push-ups, sit-ups, and jumping jacks to greet each day. Exercise oxygenates your tissues, strengthens your heart and increases your flexibility. The benefits are nearly unlimited.

If you are not exercising at all, start doing something you enjoy. It can be as simple as bouncing on a mini-trampoline for five minutes a day. If you enjoy golf, walk the course instead of taking a cart. You can take quick walks for just 15 to 20 minutes daily while pumping your arms briskly. This movement magnifies the positive effects on your heart. Even a little exercise is better than none at all!

Regular physical activity can help you prevent or manage high blood pressure. Your cholesterol levels will benefit, too. Regular physical activity boosts your "good" cholesterol while decreasing triglycerides. This one-two punch can potentially prevent the buildup of plaque in your arteries, lowering the risk of developing a heart attack or stroke. It can also help you prevent diabetes, osteoporosis, certain types of cancer and help you to maintain a healthy weight.

Need to lose some extra pounds? Exercise is a no-brainer because whenever you move your body you burn calories! The more intense the activity, the more calories you burn and the easier it is to keep your weight under control. You can lose weight by simply deciding to take the stairs instead of the elevator from now on. Walk during your lunch break. Do jumping jacks when you get sleepy during the day. Turn off the TV and go for a bike ride. Dedicated workouts are great, but any physical movement you accumulate throughout the day will help you to burn calories, too.

Want to put some zest into your sex life? Regular physical activity can leave you feeling more energized and looking better, which may have a positive effect on your sex life. But there's more to it than that. Regular physical activity can lead to enhanced arousal for women, and men who exercise regularly are less likely to have problems with erectile dysfunction than are men who don't exercise, especially as they age.

Exercise improves your mood and can you help blow off some steam after a stressful day. An energetic workout at the gym after work or over lunch can help you calm down and improve your job performance. Moving your body energetically stimulates various brain chemicals that leave you feeling happier and more relaxed than you were before you worked out. You will look better and feel better when you exercise regularly, which can boost your confidence and improve your self-esteem. It can help prevent depression and may even help you get a promotion!

Not an athlete? You don't need to be one to enjoy all the benefits of moving your body. Exercise doesn't have to be boring and can be so much fun! Be creative and consider activities such as ballroom or line dancing. Dust off your bike and find a level trail; as you gain strength and endurance, add a few hills. Have fun canoeing, gardening, playing doubles tennis or taking a water aerobics class. More vigorous exercises might include aerobic dancing, Zumba, TRX or Pilates exercise classes, biking faster than 10 miles an hour, singles tennis, jumping rope, swimming laps, uphill hiking, race walking, jogging or running.

I would like to suggest that everyone take up walking as one of the best ways to begin getting more exercise. It is low risk and easy to start. Wear a good pair of shoes and comfortable clothes. Walk as briskly as possible but so you can still carry on a conversation. Bend your elbows at a ninety-degree angle and swing them vigorously as you walk to burn more calories and increase your heart rate. As you get in better shape add hills, lengthen your stride and increase your speed. The American Heart Association recommends walking at least 30 minutes a day.

Remembering the following tips when starting an exercise program will help you achieve long-term success:

1. **Remember why you started**. People start exercising for many reasons. Remembering why you started will help keep you motivated.
2. **Do everything at your own pace**. Start off slowly and build intensity as you get stronger.

3. **Pick an exercise activity you can have fun with**. For long-term success the activity has to be something you enjoy.
4. **Do it with a friend**. If you join a fitness club or exercise with a friend you will enjoy the sessions more and be more likely to stick with it.
5. **Get a trainer**. Hiring a trainer can help hold you accountable and you will likely get faster results, too.
6. **Change it up**. Varying your exercise routine can keep you from getting bored. This is important for your motivation and also for best results.
7. **Be realistic about your goals**. Some people are motivated by goals, yet others find them stressful. If you need goals, make sure they are realistic and work towards them.

As you get a few weeks of exercise under your belt, you will be surprised by how good you feel and how good you are beginning to look! After a few more weeks your exercise routine will start to become a habit. Once this wellness secret becomes a healthy habit, you will never want to stop and it will pay you dividends for many, many years to come!

WELLNESS SECRET
7

"Avoid Drugs Whenever Possible"

We owe a tremendous debt of gratitude to the many skilled members of the medical profession who tirelessly dedicate their lives to helping the sick and saving countless lives. In addition, we are blessed to be living in times when medical advances are improving treatment and extending lives more than ever before.

American medical care is definitely the best in the world at treating disease, but in spite of all the positive benefits, its prescription medicine and surgery-based approach is not working to improve our overall health. In reality, our medical system is not really "health care" but "sickness and treatment care." Its strengths are emergency care and the treatment of disease and severe illness. Its weaknesses are disease prevention and the preservation of good health.

Spending on prescription drugs has more than doubled between 1999-2009. Prescription drug use is at an all-time high with 50 percent of American men, women and children consuming at least one prescription drug on any given day. That figure jumps for those over age 60 – when a full 90 percent in this age group have to rely on daily prescription medication! (Source-National Center for Health Statistics, Center for Disease Control and Prevention ISN 1941-4935 Sept. 2010.) We have more drugs available than ever before being prescribed in record amounts with more patients than ever taking multiple drugs at the same time. Yet we are less healthy collectively than ever before. Top it off with hospitalization and health insurance costs skyrocketing and it does not take a rocket scientist to figure out that prescription drugs and surgery are not the answer to fixing our health care crisis. The answers lie in health preservation and in preventing disease in the first place.

The prescription drug industry has a dark side that the general population rarely hears about and is seldom publicly discussed. Barbara Starfield, M.D., of the Johns Hopkins School of Hygiene and Public Health published an article in The Journal of the American Medical Association which stated that 106,000 people die annually from the "non-error, negative effects" of prescription drugs. Adverse drug events, as they are often called, occur every day across this great country of ours. These reactions are not the result of prescription errors — they routinely occur even when the correct drug is given to the correct patient in the proper dose and an unexpected reaction results that nobody anticipates.

These adverse events result in the death of patients a minimum of 106,000 times per year, and it's likely that this statistic grossly understates what many believe is a much more widespread problem. Adverse drug event statistics are poorly reported. Some estimates place the true number at nearly 500,000 deaths per year, making it a close second to cancer in the "Top 10 Causes of Death" in the U.S. Worse yet, there are an estimated 2 million more people per year who don't die yet have a violent enough reaction to prescription drugs to require hospitalization.

Medical doctors get little to no education about diet and nutrition, exercise or alternative approaches to health care. Due to the high rates of sickness and disease, their education almost out of necessity must focus on more radical chemical-based treatments and surgical interventions. That leaves the responsibility up to you as an individual to educate yourself and to make the daily decisions that will keep you healthy and out of the medical doctor's office.

I have always advocated disease prevention and maintaining good health as the antidote for prescription medication because it is far easier to keep good health than it is to reclaim your health once you have lost it.

If you are ever faced with the prospect of a serious diagnosis and a prescription drug is recommended, you should always ask the doctor the following questions:

- "Why are you prescribing this drug?"
- "What is it and how is it supposed to help?"
- "What are the possible side effects?"
- "How soon should I begin to feel better?"
- "Where can I learn more about this medication?"
- "How long must I take it?"
- "Will it react with any other medications or vitamin supplements I am already taking?"
- "What other options do I have?" and my favorite,
- "If I was your wife/husband, would you be comfortable recommending this medication to me?" Their answer to this question will sometimes surprise you!

Pharmacists are perhaps the best resource for drug information, drug-to-drug interactions, potential side effects and possible adverse reactions. It would serve you well to ask their opinion as well.

If you are currently taking medications, do not discontinue or alter how you take them in any way without first consulting your medical physician or medical specialist. Doing so can have drastic effects on your health and should never be done without direct medical supervision.

If you have chosen to begin chiropractic care or take an alternative or complimentary approach to your health challenges, your medical physician or specialist should have no problem reducing or stopping medication(s) as your health improves and warrants it. However do not take it upon yourself to make those decisions independently without their supervision. When you follow the **Seven Wellness Secrets**, you are making invaluable deposits into your "health account" in much the same way financial deposits grow in a savings account. Consistent daily choices that are constructive to your body rather than destructive will accumulate and build a reservoir of health that can be tapped into in the event you ever face a serious health problem.

Let's quickly review the **Seven Wellness Secrets**:

1. **A Healthy Spine Equals a Healthier You** –Get your spine checked by a chiropractor for spinal misalignments, get it corrected and keep it healthy with regular chiropractic checkups for optimal life-long health and wellness.

2. **Real Food Really Matters** - Make healthier food choices every day and eat more "live" constructive foods so your body has the necessary building materials to grow strong cells and naturally fight off cancer and other serious diseases before they ever start.

3. **Just Say "No" to Sweets** - Limit your intake of sugar and sweets so you stay trim, keep your immune system strong and avoid pain.

4. **Get Your Daily ZZZs** - Be sure to get adequate rest so your body is able to grow, heal properly and recharge.

5. **Stress Less** - Minimize the effects of long-term stress by first recognizing it and then taking steps to eliminate it.

6. **Keep Moving** - Keep your body moving with any and all types of exercise to maintain high levels of energy, lose extra weight and stay flexible.

7. **Avoid Drugs Whenever Possible** - Recognize the potentially serious effects of prescription medicine and always ask the right questions before starting any new medication.

More than any other factor, the health of your body determines the quality of your life. The choices you make each day determine whether you will struggle with sickness, pain, disease and exhaustion or enjoy a life full of health, wellness, peace and joy. The **Seven Wellness Secrets** are the keys to a strong, vibrant, healthy body and all of the resulting benefits. Starting with small changes is a great way to move toward a better body, better health and a better tomorrow. Put the **Seven Wellness Secrets** into action in your life today and begin to enjoy the wonderful life you deserve and have always dreamed of!

ABOUT
DR. JOHN MADEIRA

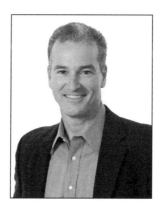

D r. John Madeira is a chiropractor and wellness expert of 30 years. He is the author of 3 books, a speaker and owner of Madeira Chiropractic Wellness Center, Inc. in Hershey, PA U.S.A. Chiropractic and natural health care changed his life as a high school football player after a neck injury caused severe migraine headaches. His passion is to see others get the health care help they need, too, so they can live a healthy, pain-free, vibrant and joy-filled life.

Madeira Chiropractic Wellness Center, Inc.
158 West Caracas Avenue
Hershey, PA 17033
MadChiroWellness.com
info@madchirowellness.com
717-533-6100

OTHER BOOKS BY
DR. JOHN MADEIRA

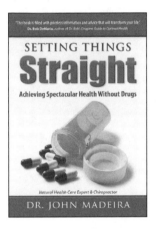

ISBN: 978-1-60725-004-3

Get ready to learn about a new and more natural approach to health care that focuses on fixing the root of the problem and not just treating symptoms with drugs. Dr. John Madeira sets things straight and reveals step by step how to enhance your body's ability to heal itself and achieve spectacular health naturally without drugs!

- Are you fed up with taking pills, dangerous side effects and exorbitant medical costs?
- Are you tired of how prescription drugs make you feel?
- Would you like natural solutions for your family's most pressing health issues?
- How much would it be worth to you to increase your energy, boost your immunity and lose weight naturally?
- Discover Dr. John's "million dollar" health habits and create your own Personal Wellness Plan!

OTHER BOOKS BY
DR. JOHN MADEIRA

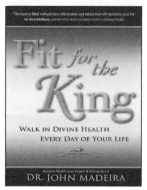

ISBN: 978-0-578-02369-4

God wants you to live an abundant life! Unfortunately too many Christians are not experiencing the quality of life that God intended. Many of God's people are suffering from pain, diseases and health disorders that are clearly preventable and correctable. Join Dr. John Madeira as he teaches simple and practical steps that will make you "Fit for the King"! Experience the joy of walking in Divine health and fulfilling your God-given destiny.

- Learn how to make Divine health a reality in your life!
- Learn the two primary reasons people get sick and die before their appointed time!
- Discover how God programmed your body to heal, protect and maintain itself!
- Learn how to experience the abundant, joy-filled life that God always intended for you!
- Enjoy a level of health that will enable you to accomplish every single assignment God planned for you!

TO ORDER:
www.PureandSimpleBooks.com
(717) 533-4840

To Order More Copies of This Book

Please Contact:
Pure and Simple Books
www.PureandSimpleBooks.com
(717) 533-4840

Quantity discounts are available